MOTHER EARTH'S EXQUISITE ELIXIR

Crystals have been used for centuries for their healing and energizing qualities. Today problems caused by overpopulation, material excess, toxic chemicals and other negative forces warrant a return to these magnificent earth-formed elements for answers. Crystals are one of Mother Earth's most exquisite answers to many of our problems because they emit healing energy on their own and can amplify and direct *our own innate remedial energy* for positive ends.

Answers to our problems in the 20th century lie within Mother Earth and her bounteous supply of healing elixirs, of which crystals are a perfect example. Through a variety of methods described in *The Truth About Crystals*, you can learn to attain the levels of awareness and understanding *vital* to a life of desired harmony and healing.

LLEWELLYN'S VANGUARD SERIES

The Truth About

CRYSTAL
HEALING

by Phyllis Galde

Author of
Crystal Healing: The Next Step
and co-author of *The Message of the Crystal Skull*

1994
Llewellyn Publications
P.O. Box 64383-360, St. Paul, MN 55164-0383
U.S.A.

First Edition
Tenth Printing, 1993
Second Edition
First Printing, 1994

International Standard Book Number:
0-87542-360-4

Cover illustration by Jyti McKie from the *Healing Earth Tarot Kit* by David and Jyti McKie

Llewellyn Publications
A Division of Llewellyn Worldwide, Ltd.
P.O. Box 64383, St. Paul, MN 55164-0383, U.S.A.

INTRODUCTION

What *is* the truth about crystal healing? How do you *really* heal with crystals? How can you best use crystal power? What value can crystals actually have for you? So many books have been written on this subject, and so many viewpoints have been presented that it's easy to become confused as to what guidelines you should follow. This helpful booklet will give you some fundamental groundwork on how to go about using crystals and benefiting from them.

Why use quartz crystals? What is it about them above all other stones that makes them so special?

Quartz crystals have been used since ancient times as powerful healing objects and meditation tools, and to make medicinal elixirs). Wise adepts have long known about their qualities and have used crystals for powerful talismans and amulets. Throughout history people have valued the beauty of quartz crystals and have used them for ornamental decoration. References to crystals are found in both the Old and New Testament, and in many other sacred teachings throughout the world.

How can minerals or stones have any influence or value? It is because there is a consciousness inherent in *all* forms of matter. Even rocks have their own consciousness! We use these crystals of the mineral kingdom to aid us in attunement with different aspects of ourselves.

Crystals have their own particular vibration of a precise and measurable intensity. This vibration attunes itself to human vibration better than any other gem or mineral. Quartz crystal is used to amplify, clarify and store energy. When you create a thought, you can amplify and clarify it by using a crystal. Quartz has long been recognized for its ability to produce electrical impulses. (Pressure on quartz crystal generates a minute electrical charge called piezoelectricity.)

You will learn how to handle and work with crystals to heal yourself, others, and the Earth. Crystals have long been revered for use in magick, for psychic development, and to see into the "hidden dimensions" that permeate physical reality. It is said that crystal has the ability to rebroadcast energy from the Universal Mind so your "inner self" can pick it up, granting you heightened perception. A crystal is a focus for this knowledge and help, and it magnifies and transmits psychic energies and healing powers.

Crystals have a hexagonal, symmetrical shape. This is a basic form in geometry, physics and atomic theory, and is a universal, perfect form in the structure of matter. The energy that radiates from clear quartz, the piezoelectric effect, amplifies healing abilities.

As a rose has been called the most perfect representation of beauty in the plant kingdom, the quartz crystal is the essence of perfection in the mineral kingdom.

HISTORICAL USES

Stories of the powers and uses of crystals and gems have come down to us from the beginning of time. Legends have it that crystal forces "set" the electromagnetic field of the Earth so that human souls could incarnate. The most popular stories dealing with the use of crystals date back to Atlantis. There, it is said, large crystals were used to generate power for cities, and it was the abuse of these energies that eventually caused the destruction of this great civilization. Edgar Cayce stated that the largest crystal generator is buried under the Atlantic Ocean near the Devil's Triangle, and this massive shift of unfocused electromagnetic energy is what causes ships and planes to go astray.

It is said that crystals were harnessed in Atlantis for power and surgery. In ancient Egypt they were the force that enabled the huge sandstone blocks to be positioned in building the pyramids. Built atop granite, the immense pressure of these stones activated the crystals found naturally in this granite, creating a gigantic generator.

Crystals were used to light the inner tunnels and chambers while the pyramids and Mystery Temples were under construction. Ancient civilizations, particularly Atlantis, used giant crystals to focus laser light. Crystals were used to fly aircraft, light homes, heal, for agriculture, and to focus beams of energy between pyramids, obelisks, temples, stone monuments and all grid points. Each pyramid amplified the energies to "light" Earth. Crystals were used to control weather, to attune initiates, and in radio waves for communicating with home bases in space (the orbiting Mother ships).

Crystals were used to generate energy, which was focused in various ways, not all of which were positive. The Atlanteans used an advanced form of hypnosis in which complex detailed visuals were projected into a person's brain, either knowingly or not. By doing this, thoughts could be influenced, as could memory banks. Near the decline of Atlantis, the dark priesthood was involved in control over others. They used crystal power to create pestilences and diseases to kill people by projecting holographically the images, fears, concepts, etc., they wanted to impress on people. They experimented on the populace. Scientists manipulated embryos to create subhuman forms to be used as slaves. Embryo development was arrested with crystal energy and hypnotic suggestion caused the embryos to stay more reptilian, scale-like. (Some people today are concerned that genetic engineering could be used for control and manipulation).

Crystal generators were built which Edgar Cayce called the "terrible crystals." Many Cayce readings refer to the use of crystals in Atlantis, both for positive and negative uses.

The author of this booklet was part of a group of individuals in Atlantis who were involved in quartz crystal experimentation on the sensations and happenings in the physical body. It was learned that much good could be accomplished in the blood and nervous systems. Unfortunately, the people in higher positions then changed the focus of her work into a more technical advancement concerning the resonating and radiating effects of crystal energy. The effects that the stone magnified were used for dominating a physical body, and the author felt that this was trespassing on the inherent rights and privacy of an individual. Finally, the author was removed entirely from the scientific department in that lifetime. This booklet, then, is an attempt to show that crystals should only be used for positive results and not to control anyone.

In Atlantis and other ancient civilizations, the Earth grid system or energy ley lines were understood and utilized. Crystals were employed to accentuate this energy grid system. Crystal energy was used as a focus for other purposes also. Atlantis and Lemuria used ultrasound and other energy forms. They used mind power by humming or "toning," and by doing so levitated rock. Crystal pyramids were used like a laser device because they could store and focus energy: sunlight energy. The crystals could encode information to a higher vibration and beam information into a person. The student could obtain the equivalent of a college education from crystal energy.

Lemurians used crystals underground to grow food because they were afraid of the giants living on the surface who were unfriendly and antagonistic. The Lemurians came to spend most of their time in caves, and so needed light energy to grow food. The stored energy from crystals was the source for this light.

In times past, crystals were used to balance harmonies in the body—to stabilize the flow of prana, to stimulate the chakras, to raise the kundalini energy. Facets of three, five, or seven were used for certain illnesses, while four- and eight-sided crystals were used to maintain balance. Crystals of various colors—red, green, blue, violet, white, etc., were used to heal various illnesses. Their healing properties restored eyesight to some in the hands of adept healers. Crystals were placed on the eyelids to draw in prana and heal organs inside the body. Much later in history, the American Indian shamans placed quartz crystals over their eyes to help them become more clairvoyant.

The ancient Greeks believed that quartz was "eternal ice" which came down from Mount Olympus, home of the Greek gods. The people used its natural magnifying power to focus the heat of the Sun's rays in order to start ceremonial fires. According to the famous Roman scholar Pliny, who wrote in the first century A.D., they used the focused crystal heat from the Sun to cauterize wounds.

The ancient Egyptians held quartz sacred, and carved drinking vessels from quartz. When they drank from these cups, the water became imbued with life-giving energy. They mined quartz, and along with many cultures began to carve it into jewelry and a variety of objects, both artistic and utilitarian.

THE CRYSTAL BALL

A booklet on crystals would be incomplete if it didn't contain at least some information on the most famous form of crystal, the crystal ball. This unique form of quartz found by archaeologists has been found in such distant areas as Peru, Siberia, Australia, Chaldea, Greece, Rome, Assyria, Persia, Japan, and China.

The ancient Chinese and Japanese regarded quartz as the perfect gem. The artists who carved spheres were thought to be the most capable of spiritual and artistic purity. They considered the quartz crystal ball the heart or "essence of the dragon," symbolic of the highest powers of creation. The Chinese and Japanese shared the term *sui ching* for quartz, which means "water essence," the source of peace and power.

Tibetan monks called crystal balls the "windows of the gods," using them as holy objects of great power. The Taoists believed that looking into the crystal's clarity "crystallized" one's being, and

they considered quartz the "gem of enlightenment."
Buddhist altars included quartz spheres as an invo-
cation of the "visible nothingness" that delineates
the duality of the material and spiritual world.

Contemplation of this "visible nothingness"
gave rise to crystal-gazing, which has been prac-
ticed since time immemorial. Crystal gazers use the
spheres as windows to faraway places, the past and
future.

AMERICAN INDIAN
LEGEND OF CRYSTALS

In ancient times, people lived in harmony with
Nature. They spoke the same language as the animals and plants. They hunted for food only to sat-
isfy their hunger and needs, always offering a
prayer of thanks for what they had taken from
Nature.

As time went on, humans lost this innocence
and harmony. They took more than they needed.
They forgot their prayers of gratitude. They killed
animals, and each other, for sport or pleasure.

The Bear Tribe, chief among the animals,
called a meeting of all the animals. They decided
that something had to be done. The Bears suggested
that they shoot back when the humans shot at them,
but the bow and arrow required too great a sacri-
fice, for one bear would have to give up his life so
that his sinew could be used for the bowstring. The

bear's claws were too long for shooting a bow anyway, and would become entangled on the string.

The Deer Tribe offered another method of dealing with the problem. One of their members said, "We will bring disease into the world. Each of us will be responsible for a different illness. When humans live out of balance with Nature, when they forget to give thanks for their food, they will get sick." And in fact the Deer did invoke rheumatism and arthritis; each animal then decided to invoke a different disease.

The Plant Tribe was more sympathetic and felt that this was too harsh a punishment, so they volunteered their help. They said that for every disease a human gets, one of them would be present to cure it. That way, if people used their intelligence, they would be able to cure their ailments and regain their balance.

All of Nature agreed to this strategy. One plant in particular spoke out. This was Tobacco, the chief of the plants. He said, "I will be the sacred herb. I will not cure any specific disease, but I will help people return to the sacred way of life, provided I am smoked or offered with prayers and ceremony. But if I am misused, if I am merely smoked for pleasure, I will cause cancer, the worst disease of all."

The close friends of the Plant Tribe, the Rock Tribe and the Mineral Tribe, agreed to help. Each mineral would have a spiritual power, a subtle vibration that could be used to regain perfect health. The Ruby, worn as an amulet, would heal the heart; the Emerald would heal the liver and eyes, and so on. The chief of the mineral tribe, Quartz Crystal, was clear, like the light of Creation itself. Quartz put his arms around his brother Tobacco and said, "I will be the sacred mineral. I will heal the mind. I will help human beings see the origin of disease. I will help to bring wisdom and clarity in dreams. And I will record their spiritual history, including our meeting today, so that in the future, if humans gaze into me, they may see their origin and the way of harmony." And so it is today.

This is a Cherokee legend, but it has been told in almost every tribe in the Americas. It tells of an ancient time of peace, a mythical homeland known to every culture on Earth. The Native Americans call it the "old way" or the "original way."

ORIGIN OF QUARTZ CRYSTAL

A crystal is a beautiful, perfect form. It contains within it harmony, balance, clarity and perfection. A quartz crystal takes over 10,000 years to form. They come from deep within the Earth's core, and were formed when the Earth was evolving. Natural quartz crystals, often referred to by ancient traditions as the "veils of the earth," frozen water or frozen light, combine the elements silicon and water through a lengthy process involving heat and pressure. They are buried in the Earth, or sometimes in streambeds where they have washed down from higher ground after being dislodged. They are often found near gold. Varieties of quartz crystal, sometimes called rock crystal, are found all over the world. The largest numbers of crystals are mined in Arkansas and Brazil.

Ninety per cent of the Earth's crust is made up of the mineral group known as silicates, a combination of silicon and oxygen, plus other elements. The simplest silicate is silicon and oxygen—quartz crystal. Chemically, it is the oxide of the element silicon, and its chemical formula is SiO_2. It has a hardness of 7 on the Mohs scale. The crystal structure of quartz is hexagonal with void spaces in geometric trails throughout the crystal.

The name crystal comes from the Greek word *crystallos* meaning "clear ice," for the ancient Greeks thought that these transparent rock crystals were in fact frozen water turned into stone. Another legend has it that Holy Water was poured out of the Heavens by God and frozen to ice in outer space on its voyage to Earth. Angels petrified the "Holy Ice" to preserve it as a protective blessing for humanity.

Quartz is the most common mineral found on the Earth. In the world of gemstones, quartz supplies more different varieties than any other mineral. Gem quartzes can be divided into three main groups: (1) crystallized quartz, (2) compact quartz, and (3) cryptocrystalline quartz.

Most crystals are formed by the repetitive addition of new matter to a growing crystalline mass. Some crystals have their origin in the magma or fiery gases of the Earth's interior or in the volcanic lava streams which reach the Earth's surface. These minerals, which include quartz, are called igneous. They are formed by the solidification of this molten mineral as it cools and hardens. As the molten rock mass cools, the atoms group together to form the essential regularity which determines the shape and composition of the crystal.

Some crystals grow from vapors in vents in volcanic regions. This type of crystal includes sulfur, and is condensed from hot mineralized gases into a solid state as the vapors are escaping from the inner Earth.

Some crystals form from water solutions or grow with the help of organisms on or near the Earth's surface. These crystals are known as sedimentary minerals, and are formed through the process of mechanical or chemical weathering. Air, water, wind and ice are the main erosion factors involved in dissolving the Earth's materials that will eventually be cemented together and occasionally crystallize.

Also, new minerals are formed by the recrystallization of existing minerals under great pressure and high temperatures in the lower regions of the Earth's crust. These metamorphic minerals undergo structural and chemical changes after the original formation, reorganizing the atoms and creating different textures, compositions and crystals.

DESCRIPTION OF CRYSTALS

A crystal is a solid material with a regular internal arrangement of atoms. Because of this orderly composition, it may form the smooth external surfaces called faces which allow us to see into the crystal when it is clear.

Most all stones are made in part of silica. The presence of this silica is what gives crystals their luminosity and crystal clearness. Crystal is brittle—as we are—and as such is a reflection of ourselves. As we shatter our being, it is seen to be rigid and crystalline in structure.

Crystals are described as being clear, milky, having rainbow prisms within, or having fractures visible along their length.

TYPES OF CRYSTALS

When people talk about crystals, they are usually referring to clear quartz, the most common form, which is often called the "grandfather" of the mineral kingdom.

Quartz crystals represent the sum total of evolution on the material plane. The six sides of the quartz crystal symbolize the six chakras, with the termination point corresponding to the crown chakra: that which connects one with the infinite.

The base of the crystal is their root or foundation with the Earth. Frequently quartz crystals are cloudy or milky at the bottom and become more clear at the top, or point. This also symbolizes a growth pattern in which the cloudiness and dullness of consciousness is cleared as one grows closer in union with the Higher Self. Within clear quartz crystals are usually found inclusions, or clouded areas. Sometimes these resemble galaxies and in a sense they are, for "As above, so below."

The most common type of clear quartz crystal is a single, six-sided length of mineral. Six natural facets join sharply together to form the terminated apex. The crystal is supported by six sides and grounds the light force at the base. These, too, are likely to be cloudy at the bottom, and clear at the top, sometimes reflecting rainbows or prisms within, with inclusions. Occasionally the crystal will be completely clear all the way through, reflecting its advanced state of growth toward perfection and complete understanding.

A quartz cluster is a natural conglomerate formation of three or more single terminated quartz crystals joined in a massive rock matrix. A quartz crystal cluster can have as many as 100 individual quartz points or terminations, or it may have only two. These clusters share a common base. They represent the evolved community, each member being individually perfect and unique, yet sharing

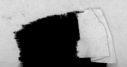

a common ground, common truth with the others. In clusters, all units join together to reap the benefits of living, learning and sharing in an advanced society. The individual crystals reflect light back and forth to one another, and all bathe in the combined radiance of the whole.

A single terminated crystal is formed when the six faces of quartz join together to form a point on one end. When *both* ends of a crystal join in this manner, a double terminated crystal is formed. These double terminated points are useful in that they have the capacity to draw in energy as well as radiate energy from either end of the crystal. By uniting the energies together in the central body of the crystal, a double terminated crystal can then project that unified essence out from both ends. These crystals are complete, and have reached a state of perfection. Instead of growing out of a hard rock surface where single terminations are formed, they grow in the center of softer clay. They know no limits or boundaries, and have grown to completion on each end. The double terminated crystals teach that it is possible to be balanced in the dual expression of spirit and matter.

A tabular crystal appears somewhat flat. This is because two of its six vertical sides are each at least twice as wide as any of the other four. This crystal may be either single or double terminated. The wide flat faces can be used as a sending and receiving board for telepathic healing and communication. It is said that these crystals are very strong and powerful. It is believed that this type of quartz crystal configuration is excellent for balancing any two elements, chakras, or people.

One more unique form of quartz crystal is the Herkimer Diamond. This is a higher vibration or octave form of crystal. These crystals are only found in one place in the world: New York. They are brilliant, usually double terminated, many with small black flecks of androxylite. Many also have rainbows. They are small but very powerful. Herkimer Diamonds are considered to be the catalysts of the quartz family. They have the potential to initiate deep inner transformation of the self.

USES OF CRYSTALS

Perhaps the greatest value of crystals is their use in healing. They have long been known for their curative effects when used in the preparation of tinctures; for their protective characteristics when worn as amulets and talismans; and for their ability to enhance the energy fields of the body as they emit uniform vibrations. They have the power of a living stone.

The energy field of this quartz, called piezo-electricity, is a major contributor to our communication systems. Computers, sonar, watches, radio stations—all use this amazing and constant, undeviating energy field. The piezo-electrical property of crystals means that they are capable of holding an electrical charge, and because of this quality, these minerals amplify healing work or meditation, which in turn speeds up the process. Quartz is the most economical source of this energy. To reduce the cost even further, laboratories are growing quartz from a slice of the real thing. It has been found that the laboratory grown specimens are the preferred kind. They are better because they are more uniform, clearer, and of a higher quality.

Crystals store and conduct energy. They can even absorb one kind of energy and emit another when squeezed, heated or cooled. Quartz crystal absorbs both magnetism from the Earth's core and radiation from the Sun, and remits that energy. Kirlian photography has recorded this energy emission, which appears in photographs as a white-light aura radiating from a blue star center. The energy radiant from clear quartz and other crystals is resonant with the human aura; this is its healing attribute.

The resonance occurs rapidly, within a few moments of holding a crystal or gemstone in the hand. Energy from crystals passes through and penetrates all matter, even into human cells. Crystal energy transmission has a magnetic polarity similar to the natural aura polarity used in laying on of hands. Its strong ability to match aura energy and resonate with it makes crystal a powerful healing tool. Clear quartz contains the greatest human resonance and the ability to transmit any color, to focus a chosen strand of its rainbow white light spectrum and use it to transmit, store, duplicate and magnify color and aura polarity.

An interesting phenomenon happens when you begin to work with crystals—for whatever reason. You will start becoming aware of an energy or force greater than what you presently contain. This force has been called your Higher Self, and it encompasses "that which you are capable of becoming. "It is your perfected self. Quartz crystals, in their wonderfully helpful way, will help you tune in to this higher aspect of yourself.

A positive act is to give a friend a quartz crystal. This helps form a link between you and him/her. It helps you to communicate psychically with that person. It is also a wonderful way to send healing energies to someone, especially if you both have similar crystals. A gilt of a crystal instills a beneficial impact in the receiver.

CRYSTALS IN HEALING

Noted healers have demonstrated that crystals can be used to accelerate bone and wound healing, relieve pain, and bring catastrophic illness into remission. Although it is said by some that there are no powers whatsoever in the crystal because it is a neutral object, its inner structure exhibits a state of perfection and balance. When a crystal is cut to the proper form, and the human mind enters into a relationship with its structural perfection, the crystal emits a vibration which extends and amplifies the powers of the healer's mind. Like a laser, it radiates energy in a coherent, highly concentrated form, and this energy may be transmitted into objects or people at will.

When people become emotionally dis tressed, a weakness forms in their subtle energy body, and disease may soon follow. With a properly attuned crystal, a healer can help release negative patterns in the energy body, allowing the physical body to return to a state of wholeness.

When healers attune their minds lovingly with a crystal, they become one with the Divine Mind, which has imprinted its consciousness in the precise, geometrical form of that structure.

Healers use crystals because the crystal is the most perfectly organized state of matter existing in nature. It is precise, regular, and free from imperfections and impurities. If people tune in to the perfection of the crystal, they can become perfect themselves.

One method of crystal healing is to tune in to the energy field of the crystal lovingly, projecting your energy into the crystal, resonating in harmony with the crystal. When you (the healer) feel the crystal is charged, scan the body of the person, being sensitive to areas of obvious imbalance where healing energies should be directed. A good focal point is the heart chakra, where through visualization the problems intuitively felt can be brought to awareness. Then snap the crystal, like a whip cracking (by flicking the wrist and hand holding the crystal), releasing the negativity that was held in the subtle body.

The crystal can take the feeling of love in the healer's heart and amplify it so a concentrated stream of energy is emitted from the crystal for use in healing. This amplified energy field can help persons dislodge inhibitions which block the flow for their higher life energies.

The crystal works in much the same way that a laser does: It takes scattered rays of energy and focuses them. It makes the energy field coherent and unidirectional so that a tremendous force is generated. When used with love, the crystal unites the energies of the mind. It brings these energies into a pattern, exactly fitting the life energies of the person seeking to be healed, and then amplifies them for the healing.

To use the crystal effectively, it is necessary to turn off the rational mind, so you may enter a right-brain meditative state and intuitively tune into the energies focused by the crystal transmitter.

There are many methods of uses for crystal healing. Perhaps the best advice to follow is to listen to your own intuition. Use what works best for you. Practice on yourself and people close to you. Meditate and listen to what the voice within gently suggests to you.

The general size of crystal to use for healing is whatever fits comfortably in the palm of your hand, or, what you are attracted to use. Its size is not so important as the feel or *essence* of it. It isn't necessary to have a large piece of quartz; a small piece will suffice in most cases.

Some possible methods for healing are to place crystals or gemstones on the seven main chakra points. Place a crystal anywhere on the body where there is a pain or discomfort. Also, a crystal can be held near the source of pain and rotated in a clockwise motion to draw out the problem. Snap the crystal to get rid of the unwelcome vibrations. Single crystals can be placed near the soles of the feet and the palms of the hands to draw out blocks and balance energies.

Crystals are excellent biofeedback tools, and work well with creative visualization for mood and body changes. When feeling cold or chilled, hold a crystal in the left hand and draw warmth. Do this in a color meditation with deep breathing, drawing in the energy—visualized as the color red—through the left side of the body, in a circuit coursing through the body that releases it from the right side to the Earth or sky. Continue doing this for several minutes until you feel warm. This works for cooling with blue as well.

For cheering, draw yellow in the same way; for calming, draw violet or indigo. Body metabolism and heart rate can be raised or lowered by this, an effect already familiar to those who have used deep breathing.

Use crystals in visualizations, affirmations, and rituals to amplify and intensify what is being done. Generally, use a crystal in the left hand to receive energy, and in the right hand to send it, but this can be opposite in some people. Experiment and learn what works best.

Crystals can relieve pain almost magickally. In another self-healing exercise, hold a crystal in the left hand, feel the energy polarity build from it; place the right hand gently on a pain area and hold it there. The pain is usually gone within half an hour.

A different method recommends that you set the crystal directly on the pain area; hold it flat in the palm of the hand with the thumb; or grip it between the fingers, pointing downward. When you remove the crystal, the pain goes away.

Crystals can be used effectively in aura reading and aura healing. Hold a crystal in whichever hand feels correct, and scan the aura of the person from the head down to the toes. Feel for heat, tingling, cold, resistance. When you encounter these, rotate the crystal counterclockwise and touch the tip to the area. This energizes the aura. A clockwise motion takes energy out. After you have gone down the front and the back of the person, brush down the aura to cleanse and seal the chakras.

CHOOSING A CRYSTAL

How do you choose a crystal that's right for you? How do you know which one will help you? Listen to your inner self, and select the crystal that's interesting and attractive to you.

The best way is to handle and hold it, being sensitive to how it feels. Appearance is secondary. Pick a stone by attraction, by being drawn to touch it, then hold it in the left hand loosely. Let it rest against the palm chakra and notice the impressions, colors, sounds, and mood feelings that accompany the stone. No two crystals are the same; they are like snowflakes. Each will resonate differently. Look for one that will resonate with *your* being, regardless of size, shape, color, clarity, or jeweler's quality. It's the subtle polarity impression which is important. The crystal should feel alive in the hand, vibrate, or radiate—it should feel good. A tiny quartz no larger than a thumbnail can be powerful and effective. Look for pleasing colors, unchipped points, and symmetrical shapes, but these appearances are secondary to the energy vibrations. Crystals are like cats in that *they* select their owner. If you are supposed to have a particular crystal, it will come to you.

If you want to check out the energy of a crystal, here's an interesting technique. Wait until you feel quiet and centered in your heart, then hold the crystal in your left hand. Curl your tongue so that its tip touches the middle-back of your mouth. This area joins the energy of your two major acupuncture meridians and increases your sensitivity. You may feel the crystal activate an organ, a chakra, a part of the body. You may feel a shift in consciousness, or simply feel warmth or tingling in your hand. Give it a few minutes to speak to you in its own way.

CRYSTAL CLEANSING

There are many different viewpoints on crystal cleansing, and whether it's even necessary or not. Follow your own feelings/intuitions on this. If you do feel your crystal needs cleansing, then it probably does. Here are some suggested methods of cleansing and clearing crystals. Use whatever feels right for you.

Use spring water and mix salt in it; preferably sea salt. Use a teaspoon to a tablespoon in a cup or more of water. Let the crystal soak overnight. Some say that salt is too harsh, and it removes energy, but is all right to use on a crystal that has much negativity attached to it. Others say that salt seals the crystal and traps the energy within it. It's just like swimming in salt water—it leaves your skin coated, but swimming in fresh water leaves you feeling refreshed and exhilarated.

You can run cold water over the crystal to cleanse it, as will just holding it in your hands visualizing it being cleansed by light, or by Niagara Falls. Crystals love to be out in the sunlight, because they are radiant energy sources. This is an excellent way to restore their energy. You owe it to your stones to give them some Sun! You can clear crystals by resting them in rose petals. The rose essence strips only the negativity from the crystals.

If you have a piece which has a particularly strong charge that you want to get rid of, bury it in the moist ground. If you live in the desert, water the immediate area it's buried under. Give the crystal a week or two (minimum of three days) to ground out.

When you dip or soak your crystal in water, bless the water. This will transform its energies into usefulness and thanks before you pour the water on a plant or onto the Earth.

CRYSTALS IN MEDITATION

Quartz crystals are an aid in meditation, as they have the ability to cut through confusion and help you tune into your Higher Self.

Take a cleansed crystal and "charge" it by centering yourself; then hold the crystal to your third eye. Program it with the purpose you wish to achieve. You can charge your crystal by focusing your desires into the luminous perfection of the crystal. When energy passes through a quartz crystal it becomes harmonized, and the natural balance is preserved. In practical terms, if the energies of the crystal user are not in balance, there will be a natural tendency of the crystal to correct and rebalance any energies that a person transmits through the crystal.

The natural tendency of the mineral kingdom is to create perfect balance and harmony. This elemental energy is largely directed by our Higher Will. We need only to tune into that Higher Self to live in harmony with ourselves, others and the world.

Use your crystal to help you achieve an altered state of mind to access information which you otherwise wouldn't know. Use the crystal as a focusing device to reach a quiet, meditative state. This altered state of awareness, sometimes called a trance state, allows you to delve deeply into the stored material of your subconscious to answer questions or to gain information. This trance state can also sensitize you to certain etheric vibrations so you can "see" the future or past.

CRYSTAL POWER

Crystals have a history of capturing people's imaginations. The crystal structures are aesthetically pleasing as well as precise, implying an order to the universe that is reassuring to the pattern-seeking human mind. But crystals are more than beautiful examples of the order of the universe. Crystal power amplifies universal forces that can be used to modify, accumulate and direct the powerful mental, psychic and material energies of being.

The book *Crystal Power* by Michael G. Smith contains instructions on how to build crystal devices to heal, direct energies, communicate with entities from other worlds, travel through time and the astral planes, and more. Why would using these crystal devices benefit you?

What you think is what you get. You're probably familiar with most of the positive thinking procedures and how they apply to your life. They *always* work. The only difference is how fast or how slowly they work. With the use of the crystal devices explained in *Crystal Power*, you can learn how to cut down on time and effort. Your time is important! Also, the devices amplify your intent many times over.

The first tool you can learn to make is an *Atlantean Power Rod*. One of the most valuable uses for this type of rod is in healing, where the energy from the rod is used to remove energy blockages in the biomagnetic field of the body. This provides a balanced flow of the body's life-force energy. Removing the energy blocks provides a balance, while the body actually does the healing itself. This type of healing is easily done with plants, animals and people.

Anyone can learn to construct an Atlantean Power Rod in a short time with some simple materials. The energy used is natural and basic to life; the technique of operation is simple.

Very likely people will need to take responsibility for self-healing and for solving problems in the near future. Many people are already taking constructive action regarding their own health. After all, we're breathing poisonous gas for air, drinking impure water, and eating contaminated food as a result of our present society. Many people are suffering from mental, emotional, spiritual, and physical disorders and diseases. This is even more disturbing when we realize that most of the disorders come from a social order and environment that we have created ourselves.

In the area of health and healing, all diseases become curable. The use of these wands employing crystal energy is actually a simple process that allows the balance of the body to be restored. The affected organism heals itself.

The Atlantean Power Rod contains the very essence of ancient advanced science. The basic rod is a hollow copper tube with a copper cap at one end. At the other end is a quartz crystal, which is about ¾" to 1" in diameter. It is about 1 ½" to 3" long. The tip of the crystal should have clear, unchipped facets at its point (the six-sided point of the crystal). The outer covering or insulation is leather, wrapped in a flat spiral. Some healing wands have quartz crystal in both ends and others have just one crystal with a copper end cap at the other end.

The copper tube acts as an energy accumulater, or funnel; the leather is an insulator, and the quartz crystal acts as an energy transducer, capacitor, and focus for the beam of energy. The only thing that moves through an energy wand is energy. It operates in the exact degree of power and efficiency as the operator it is attuned to. As soon as construction is complete, it begins functioning in the passive mode, radiating energy in all directions from the crystal. Picked up by the operator, it continues to function in this manner. When the operator focuses it by pointing and thinking/visualizing, a blue-white ray of energy beams in that direction from the point of the quartz crystal at the end. Thought switches the device from passive radiating energy to an active energy beam. Intensity and distance of the beam are determined by a combination of thoughts amplified by the emotions of the individual operator.

These machines are capable of delivering a large amount of accurately focused energy at short or long distances with little or no time delay involved. The operator does not have to move or travel to affect its usage. These crystal energy tools, in the hands of an experienced operator, have the ability to reach out through space and time, transforming both energy and matter on a subatomic level. Transforming radioactive substances into harmless elements is now possible, as is removing other harmful substances like poison chemicals, dirty air, contaminated food and water, even the Earth itself. These transmutations are completely natural processes. The Earth *will* disperse, transform, and purify itself over a long period of time; these devices merely speed up normal processes.

The Crystal Power Rod is in actuality a miniature linear accelerator. It is a 12" long subatomic particle beam generator. These are just smaller versions of the most powerful machines ever constructed. Many sub-atomic particles travel at nearly the speed of light. They also travel through all materials: Earth, wood, metal, concrete, and deep space.

Many people feel an intuitive familiarity with these energy wands. Some say it may be from a previous incarnation in one of the ancient civilizations of Earth, or even another lifetime on another planet. It may be from references in ancient writings, or even present day UFO reports. Many engineers and researchers agree that as advances in sophistication are made, machines become simpler instead of more complex. This is obviously the case with crystal devices, and mind/ particle machines. They are in balance with universal laws and physics, being both sensible and practical. The fundamental application is balance and healing, whether applied to people, plants, animals, poisoned air, polluted foods, contaminated water, or our chemically and radioactively suffering Earth Mother. Overall balance and total healing is a top priority for many of us in this lifetime.

Another incredible crystal device to make is an *Atlantean Crystal Headband*. The Headband is a relatively simple device with no moving parts. It is composed of a copper band with a silver disc and a clear-tipped quartz crystal on top of the silver disc. Complete instructions may be found in the book *Crystal Power* offered through Llewellyn.

The Atlantean Crystal is regarded as a device with the ability to amplify thoughts. It focuses and beams these thoughts to a specific destination, depending on the wishes of the operator. The quartz crystal, in conjunction with the copper band and silver disc, acts as a capacitor for storing the energy and a transducer for changing its form. Thoughts and images are converted at the speed of light into beams, which are sent to a receiver at some distance or time. The receiver converts the stream of particles back into images, thoughts and emotions.

This is similar to the principles involved in radio and television, except the machine is simpler and more sophisticated, with an increased number of the energy workings dependent on the individual and naturally occurring particle fields.

This device augments psychic impressions. In many cases, this can be extremely helpful. A few things to be aware of are that it will amplify *all* emotions and thoughts inside you. Some of these may not be the thoughts you had planned on using, so until you become adept at its use, make sure you adopt a very positive attitude when using the Crystal Headband. It is helpful to have your thoughts focused and be in a pleasing frame of mind when first learning to use this device.

Another helpful crystal tool is the *Crystal Space/time Communications Generator*. The crystal space/time generator also functions as a super shield/force field for the home. This is a side effect you can make use of when the communications generator is not being used as a communication unit.

A group of people are sitting in a circle in a living room. In the middle of the circle on the carpet is a shiny copper disc, about one foot in diameter. Centered on the disc is a large quartz crystal, nearly seven inches high, four inches in diameter, and mounted in a round copper cylinder like a cup. The sharp point of the crystal is almost clear as it reflects light like a prism, breaking it into the colors of the rainbow.

The people sit quietly, connecting the circle by joining hands and visualizing a blue-white light beacon emanating from the tip of the power crystal, beaming out into space. Their project is to attempt to communicate with star people, and in the process they are learning much about themselves. You, too, can work with other like-minded people to communicate with helpful beings from other spaces and times with this crystal communications generator.

Not only is this unit an attractive looking display unit to adorn your home, but it can be mentally programmed to project a blue-white light force-field dome over and around your house. After it's set in place, think of it radiating energy in all directions, and visualize the energy dome forming. Charge it with a desire for protection of your home, and leave it as such for as long as you want.

The *Home and Garden Field Projector* will protect your home and land from unwanted thought influences, UHF and VHF waves, etc., which can disturb your peace of mind. It will also keep insects and unwanted visitors away from your garden. This crystal instrument is simple and economical to build and use. It can be constructed from materials left over from earlier experiments. See *Crystal Power* for complete instructions and list of supplies needed.

A double terminated quartz crystal can be used as an energy shield. Remember that a quartz crystal is a transducer and capacitor for energy. It will store and change energy from one kind to another. By keeping a double terminated crystal close to your body over a period of time, it will tune itself to your conscious and biomagnetic field. You can speed up this process by thinking about and visualizing a white circle of protection around yourself, and emotionally charging the crystal to the best of your ability. Keep your crystal close to you at all times. Keep it in your pocket, your purse, or at least in your house. When you travel, it should go with you.

This type of quartz crystal should have clear points with unchipped facets. It has a six-sided point at each end or termination. Size can vary from an inch to several inches long. Try to find one that is clear and perfectly formed. This Energy Shield Crystal will augment your blue-white light shield, and protect you against any unwholesome thought influences and vibrations coming at you.

The *Double Terminated Quartz Crystal Shield* can protect you 24 hours a day. In an average day an unprotected person is subjected to all types of radiation (from nuclear to electronic), from electrical systems, germ warfare, toxic agents, radio waves, microwaves, solar and stellar radiation, low frequency waves used by governments, and more. We live in a vast sea of radiation of all types. Sensitive people sometimes find this to be disturbing and offensive. This double terminated quartz is a useful tool for people who need to work calmly and undisturbed in their daily lives.

Unfortunately, we are presently living in a world of chaos. As this chaos increases (since it's composed of electromagnetic disturbances), psionic subatomic machines are easier to use. As the Earth's fields become more disturbed, these crystal machines work more quickly. The harder it becomes for obsolete systems to work, the easier it becomes for the new systems to operate. Use of crystals will become popular and necessary. If you *haven't* experimented with crystal power and crystal energy already, you are missing out on some valuable assistance from our friends in the mineral kingdom. You owe it to yourself to become acquainted with this simple, inexpensive form of energy.

CRYSTALS FOR PSYCHIC/SPIRITUAL DEVELOPMENT

It is helpful to use quartz crystal as a tool for clear channeling of your higher self into your ordinary life. Recall that a crystal is an individual source of perfect form, each with its own frequency of vibration for focusing your positive thought-forms.

Crystals help us in becoming more complete, in taking more responsibility for our actions, and they guide our footsteps on the path to spiritual awakening. They lovingly help us build a greater harmony of mind and spirit to become the radiant beings that we all are.

The physical body is composed mostly of silica, and we all need supplements of this to make up for the silica which is depleted. Quartz crystal, remember, is composed of silicon dioxide. Silica equalizes psychic energy forces in the body so the kundalini energy may rise safely and open the third eye. The New Age person will need *more* silica in their form. They will need the stimulation of the "sand crystals" in the pineal gland to better understand communications from the Forces of Light.

Meditation and prayer create powerful rays of White Light, which is like food for the soul. This White Light stimulates the pineal gland and the crystals of silica of which it is composed. Holding a crystal in the left hand during meditation steps up the frequencies and energies for the pineal gland (third eye). A small crystal taped on the forehead over the third eye is a powerful charger when meditating.

The silica found in our bodies is in the form of crystals. This silica in the connective tissues bind the body cells together. Silica is a prominent part of brain tissues also. The brain is filled with "dust'" crystal. These infinitesimal dust crystals are found in all the brain cells, especially in the third eye area, the pineal gland.

Focused gazing or meditation on a quartz crystal can stimulate the pineal crystals, through the eye ray, bringing about development of clairvoyance, clairaudience, and clairsentience. To develop clairaudient perception, hold a crystal in your hand and combine its power with chanting. Each crystal holds within its structure a sacred code of sound peculiar to it alone. This sound can be discerned by chanting and focusing attention upon the crystal you have chosen.

In the great Temples of Initiation, the secret password was encoded in quartz crystal. The person seeking initiation would have to hear the password clairvoyantly from a spirit guardian before they would be able to enter. The right vibration or sound would automatically open the portal, much as our automatic door openers work now with light breaking a barrier.

Another way in which crystals help your spiritual progress is by their rainbow light. Attach a string to your crystal and hang it in the window so the sunlight shining through it will shower you with the colors of the rainbow. Sit in this prism of rainbow light if you can. Otherwise, visualize the light rays coming through your crystal. This light will stimulate your etheric body and increase your auric protection against adverse influences, and raise your level of consciousness.

Quartz crystals represent crystallized energies of Sun and light frequencies. An average person is like a walking crystal antenna who is out of tune! You can fine-tune *your* body and bloodstream, much like harmonizing a song or tuning a violin, using the energies of crystals.

CRYSTALS AND PYRAMIDS

Tiny crystals shaped like pyramids are floating throughout the bloodstream, bearing the DNA code of the individual soul. Throughout the universe, the pyramid is known as the principle geometric form for matter and consciousness. Hydrogen atoms contain pryamidal units. All matter is made up of hydrogen.

The Great Pyramid in Egypt symbolizes the gateway on Earth through which we will attain a higher plateau of evolution. Pyramids are built on grid formations, and pyramids and crystals can focus energies on these lines. Even on other planets throughout the solar system, pyramids are built as a focus of energy (we have pictures of pyramids on Mars, courtesy of the space program). Each pyramid is connected to cosmic chronomonitors which measure the vibratory levels of consciousness on a planet in units of 1000 years.

CRYSTAL LEARNING

The quartz crystal can be a wonderful help in helping you to learn new information. The crystal is able to process information holographically, as compared to the computer, which stores and retrieves information bit by bit.

Ancient people, especially in Atlantis, used the crystal for storing information. It stores and retrieves knowledge as whole, intact images which don't need to be converted into parts, as does the electronic computer. Ancient scientists, and seers, could mentally project their knowledge, whole and complete, into the natural micro-computer field of a crystal. Whenever they needed to retrieve their information, they attuned themselves to the crystal, and the stored images were converted into the original concepts.

In today's world of learning, a mind/crystal interface is an interesting possibility. A student can learn math, art, science, etc., with his "crystal computer." The crystal computer will have a program of stored-image subjects. When the student tunes in to the computer and becomes "at one" with it, easily processing huge amounts of information both instantaneously and holographically. After knowing things from the inside, the next task is to translate that knowledge from the right brain into the logical left brain which processes knowledge verbally.

FUTURE USE OF CRYSTALS

It is said that there are 12 crystalline fields of communication within the Earth. Future generations will be able to communicate with the distant galaxies, and perhaps even crystals for this communication. These 12 crystalline fields will be discovered throughout the world in subterranean tunnels or channels where crystal energy has been previously used to outfit a scientific technology. This crystalline network is a system of channels which connect with resonating crystalline structures for image and information processing. There are grid mappings that are presently not understood, but which will be used as coordination points for many fields of communication to overlap with the living Light in the universe. These 12 grids act as focal points for the transmission of faster-than-light particles. Crystal communication is capable of going beyond our electromagnetic spectrum by being activated by the proper psi grids aligned with the 12 crystalline chambers built into the grid structure of the Earth. Astronomers will use this crystal latticework to bend the light waves for universal communication.

CRYSTAL COUSINS

There are many other gemstones besides clear quartz crystal which can be enjoyable and beneficial. Many different types of beautifully polished gemstones which can be used for healing meditation, energy and enjoyment.

Gems come in many different colors, sizes, shapes, and varieties. Their material existence is also shown by their weight, hardness, and chemical composition. Their psychic or spiritual influence is shown to us by the inner geometric construction and vibrations; the shape and mathematical relationship of their crystals.

Nearly all gemstones are crystalline in structure. There are only a few which are not. Amber is fossilized tree sap. Coral is created by an underwater creature, and pearls are secretions. Opal is a member of the quartz group, but it lacks a crystal structure and is still in a comparatively watery state. Gemstones have a symmetry, and it is their relationship to the light which passes through them which makes them so valuable for our well-being.

Some gemstones are radiant, and some are receptive. General colors which are radiant include red: ruby, garnet, amethyst, etc. They will help you change your world. They are creative and expansive. The receptive stones are magnetic and help you to absorb what you need. They help manifest what you visualize, and draw your ideas into form. They have a feminine quality. Moonstones are receptive, as are green, black, or any dark stones. The softer stones are receptive. A few stones are receptive and radiant at the same time, like topaz.

WHAT STONES TO USE?

There have been basic guidelines throughout history which recommend what stones to use for a given situation, but it is always best to listen to your own intuition. The stone or color you are attracted to at a given time has the vibrations your body needs for energy or balancing. When you begin to listen to your "sixth sense," your intuition, most likely it's your Higher Self speaking to you through inner channels. You may be drawn to a particular stone—attracted to it, desire to have it or wear it. You probably need what that stone has to offer; the information it has to give to you. Listen to what your body is telling you. You are intuitively sensing the vibration of that particular stone and its effect on your personal energy pattern or being.

There is a great "truth detector" that your body has built into it. If you read/learn/hear/see something which you believe to be true, something that strikes a chord and rings true with your Higher Self, you will feel chills coursing through your body ("goose bumps"). This feeling is fleeting, and you must be still within to be aware of it. Know that this feeling accompanies a revelation of "truth" for you. If a gemstone elicits this feeling in you, listen to what the stone is telling you.

An excellent addition to have in your collection is a lodestone. This is a very inexpensive stone, and is valuable to have because it has the ability to *balance* the energies of your other stones, and it helps to focus their beneficial aspects. The different stones or crystals can then work together in a more cohesive manner.

Following is a listing of the magnificently polished gemstones, along with descriptions of them, their qualities and some of their uses. Among other things, they have been used for healing, well-being, energy and good luck. Each stone has its special energies, its unique qualities and vibrations indigenous to its place of origin. They freely share their special gifts and energies with you.

AMAZONITE

Amazonite is a light, aqua-green stone with white mottled flecks. The rock typically originates from the New England States and Colorado. It is composed of potassium feldspar, and is a green variety of microline. The name is derived from amazon-stone, from the Amazon River. While amazonite is found in Brazil, it is not found by the Amazon River!

It is a sacred stone highly valued and used extensively by the ancient Egyptians. Amazonite is cooling and soothing to your mental state. This stone is important for healing and spiritual growth. It helps to align the heart and solar plexus chakras. It also aligns the etheric and mental bodies. As a thought amplifier, amazonite magnifies the consciousness stored in these chakras, especially the psychological attributes.

This pleasing, calming stone makes it easier for the life force to act as a bonding agent and this penetrates to the molecular level. It's an enhancer for most other vibrational remedies. On the cellular level, the brain processes are stimulated. All the body energy currents are strengthened by amazonite.

AMETHYST

Amethyst is a regal violet gemstone with whitish stripes. The purple color comes from the presence of manganese during its formation. It is a form of crystallized quartz, composed of silica. It is found mostly in Brazil.

Amethyst is a radiant gemstone, meaning that its energies are expansive. It is said that when you meditate with amethyst you are helping the Earth, because the violet ray will help to transform the entire world into a better place. It is the most highly valued stone in the quartz group. It has many supernatural powers. It is said to bring luck, ensure constancy, protect against magic and homesickness. It has long been known to help against drunkenness.

Violet has a calming effect upon the nervous system. Insomnia may be relieved by gently rubbing an amethyst on the temples or forehead, and can be used for tension and migraine headaches. It is one of the best to use for meditation. It is here to teach the lesson of humility, to "Let go and let God." Amethyst is very useful for people grieving over lost loved ones, as it subliminally communicates that there is no death. Amethyst is recommended for stimulating greater love, and attunement for healing forces. In directing the energy of the amethyst to the lungs, relief may be obtained for asthma and circulation problems. You can recharge your own energy by holding an amethyst over the crown chakra, third eye, or heart chakra. A very high vibration centered in love, balance, and harmony will be transferred.

APACHE TEAR DROP

Apache tear drop is a form of black obsidian. It is a calming translucent stone, found in Arizona and other parts of the U.S. It is composed of feldspar, hornblend, biotite and quartz. It was formed by rhythmic crystallization which produces a separation of light and dark materials into spherical shapes, and is a form of volcanic glass.

There is a haunting legend about the Apache tear drop. After the Pinal Apaches had made several raids on a settlement in Arizona, the military regulars and some volunteers trailed the tracks of the stolen cattle and waited for dawn to attack the Apaches. The Apaches, confident in the safety of their location, were completely surprised and outnumbered in the attack. Nearly 50 of the band of 75 Apaches were killed in the first volley of shots. The rest of the tribe retreated to the cliff's edge and chose death by leaping over the edge rather than die at the hands of the white men.

For years afterward those who ventured up the treacherous face of Big Pacacho in Arizona found skeletons, or could see the bleached bones wedged in the crevices of the side of the cliff.

The Apache squaws and the lovers of those who had died gathered a short distance from the base of the cliff where the sands were white, and for a moon they wept for their dead. They mourned greatly, for they realized that not only had their 75 brave Apache warriors died, but with them had died the great fighting spirit of the Pinal Apaches.

Their sadness was so great, and their burden of sorrow so sincere that the Great Father imbedded into black stones the tears of the Apache women who mourned their dead. These black obsidian stones, when held to the light, reveal the translucent tear of the Apache. The stones bring good luck to those possessing them. It is said that whoever owns an Apache tear drop will never have to cry again, for the Apache maidens have shed their tears in place of yours.

The Apache tear drops are also said to balance the emotional nature and protect one from being taken advantage of. It can be carried as an amulet to stimulate success in business endeavors. It is also used to produce clear vision and to increase psychic powers.

Black obsidian is a powerful meditation stone. The purpose of this gemstone is to bring to light that which is hidden from the conscious mind. It dissolves suppressed negative patterns and purifies them. It *can* create a somewhat radical behavior change as new positive attitudes replace old, negative, egocentric patterns.

AVENTURINE

Aventurine is a pleasing dark green stone with a metallic iridescence or spangled appearance. It is a compact quartz stone, composed of silica with some impurities. It is found in India, China and Brazil.

It is said to bring luck and adventures in love and games. It makes an individual independent and original. It has a binding and healing force, and is good for skin diseases and improving the complexion. At one time it was used to cure nearsightedness. It is helpful for the etheric, emotional and mental bodies. Aventurine has strong healing energies, and affects the pituitary gland. It can be used for creative visualization, higher-self attunement, and is good for the muscle and nervous system.

Aventurine is a good stone for artists, writers and all those of a creative nature. It brings prosperity; the green vibrations attract money.

BLOODSTONE

Bloodstone is a green, opaque stone with spotted red flecks. It is a member of the cryptocrystalline quartz group, and is composed of silica. Bloodstone belongs to the general group of chalcedony and is found in India, Australia, Brazil, China and the U.S.

Bloodstone contains deep earth-green and a deep, blood red. Together these create a powerful cleanser for the physical body. It is an important purifier for the kidneys, liver, spleen and blood. In times past, bloodstone was used to stop bleeding and hemorrhage by wounded soldiers and mothers-to-be. It will detoxify the body. Bloodstone helps transform the body to enable it to carry more light and energy.

Legend has it that when Christ was crucified, the blood from his wound dripped to the green jasper ground, spotting it red and thus forming this stone. This stone was also known as heliotrope, and it was believed that if one covered the stone with the herb heliotrope, the owner became invisible. This combination was used in many other magical rites also.

BLUE LACE AGATE

Blue lace agate is a beautiful, pale sky blue stone with concentric markings. It is a cryptocrystalline quartz stone. Agate is a banded chalcedony, the bands having been formed by rhythmic crystallization. Agates are found as nodules or geodes in siliceous volcanic rocks. This stone comes from southwest Africa.

Agate strengthens the power of the Sun in your astrological sign when you wear it. It helps you stay well-balanced. It sharpens the sight, illuminates the mind and helps you speak.

Blue lace agate helps you develop and realize your inner peace. These stones affect the physical body, first at the densest levels, and then at the levels of some of the higher bodies as well.

CARNELIAN

Carnelian is a translucent orange-red stone. It is a cryptocrystalline quartz, composed of silica. It is found in India and South America.

In ancient times carnelian was thought to still the blood and soften anger. It is a gem of the Earth, a symbol of the strength and beauty of our planet.

It is good for people who are absent minded, confused or unfocused. It strengthens the voice and helps one become more eloquent and charitable. Carnelian carries the stories and records of our Earth and can be used to see into the past. This stone symbolizes good luck and contentment.

This gem does good things to the body just by wearing it, as it feeds energy molecules directly through the skin, just as one can breathe in prana by inhaling air. Carnelian is one of the few gems that harmonizes effectively with the elements of fire and earth today. It helps cleanse the liver if you hold the stone over the liver and massage the area.

CRAZY LACE AGATE

Crazy lace agate, also known as Mexican agate, is an attractive, white, opaque stone, patterned like a beautiful, multicolored paisley cloth. It is a cryptocrystalline quartz, found in Mexico.

In ancient times, this agate was worn to placate the gods, and to give courage. It will sharpen your sight, help the eyes, illuminate your mind, allow you to be more eloquent and give vitality. It keeps the wearer well-balanced and serious. Lace agate strengthens the Sun in its wearer, and improves the ego and self-esteem. It gives you a feeling of consolation despite the hardships of life. It has been considered symbolical of the third eye, and the symbol of the spiritual love of good. It helps to banish fear. It is a good general healing stone.

JADE

Jade is a soothing green color. It is an avocado green gem, with darker mottled flecks of green in it. This variety of jade comes from Wyoming. It is composed of sodium aluminum silicate, and because of its felt-like structure, it is very tough and resistant.

The name goes back to the time of the Spanish conquest of Central and South America and means *piedra de ijada* (hip stone), as it was used as a protection against and cure for kidney diseases. Jade is the prince of peace and tranquillity. It acts quietly as a consciousness raiser of human development. It dispels negativity by the constant emission of soothing and cleaning vibrations.

It is said that jade is not from the Earth, but is a mutation from a planet outside this solar system. Jade can never harm anyone wearing it, for it does not absorb negative attributes of any nature. It is said to prolong life, protect one from accidents, and quiet inner restlessness.

MOONSTONE

Moonstone is a translucent, light toned gem of many hues, or else is colorless, with a milky-blue sheen. It is the most important gemstone of the feldspar group. It is composed of potassium feldspar. Feldspars are silicates of aluminum and either potassium, sodium or calcium. It comes from Ceylon or Brazil.

Moonstone is a receptive stone. It helps you to balance and soothe your emotions so you don't have to react from an emotional state. It helps your Higher Self control your emotions so you can grow more spiritually. Moonstones help you experience calmness and peace of mind.

These stones help women's hormonal and emotional equilibrium, and they help men become more in tune with the feminine side of themselves. The moonstone can act as a magical link so that your guides can communicate with you easier to know what your life path really is. The moonstone can hold charges in it, and may need to be cleansed occasionally.

PETRIFIED WOOD

Petrified wood, also known as fossilized wood, is a gray-brown conglomerate of muted tones. It can have light brown, yellow, red, pink, and even blue to violet colors in it. It is a microcrystalline quartz and a member of the chalcedony family. The organic wood is not really changed into stone, only the shape and structural elements of the wood are preserved. It is found mainly in the southwest U.S.

Petrified wood is very earthy, and will assist you in becoming grounded and balanced. If you feel spacey and not quite "with it", having a piece of petrified wood near you will restore your subtle bodies to a more harmonious grounded state, and you will be able to think and reason more clearly.

It was used by the American Indians as a protective amulet against accidents, injuries and infections. It was thought to bring good luck, build reserves of physical energy, help ease mental and emotional stress, and encourage emotional security.

This stone is helpful for arthritis, environmental pollutants, skeletal systems, enhances longevity and generally strengthens the body.

RHODONITE

Rhodonite is an attractive rose pink stone with black veinings. It is composed of manganese metasilicate. The name comes from its color (Greek for rose). It is found in Canada, Mexico, and the U.S.

Rhodonite is good for mental unrest and confusion, anxious forebodings and incoherence. It fends off unwanted influences from the etheric planes. It is good for psychically sensitive people who would prefer to be left in peace. It relieves anxiety, stress, promotes mental balance, and mental clarity. Rhodonite helps one deal with sensitivity, self-esteem, and become more self-confident. On the physical level, it is good for the skeletal system.

ROSE QUARTZ

Rose quartz is a gentle, pale to medium pink translucent form of quartz. It comes from Brazil. This stone has a soft and useful frequency, and does not conflict with any other stones. It is an important stone for the heart chakra, and for giving and receiving love. It helps to dissolve all burdens and traumas that have burdened the heart. Rose quartz assists in understanding and dissolving problems so the heart is better able to know love. As its presence is felt by the body, sorrows, fears, and resentments are replaced by a sense of personal fulfillment and peace.

This stone promotes the vibrations of universal love and inner serenity. It teaches that the many negative childhood experiences enable the self to learn how to love and nurture itself. It also enlivens the imagination to be able to create beautiful forms.

RUTILATED QUARTZ

Rutilated quartz is clear quartz with threads of titanium dioxide (gold filaments) running through it. Much of this stone comes from Brazil. It is also called needle stone, or angel's hair.

Rutilated quartz energizes, rejuvenates, and balances the system. It raises your vibrations, increases clairvoyance, and strengthens thought projections. This gemstone helps the body in the assimilation of nutrients, helps the immune system function more effectively, slows diseases of aging, and prevents depression.

The crossing of the rutiles in this type of quartz represents the accord of tissue regeneration within the physical body. This mineral also stimulates the electrical properties of the body.

SMOKY QUARTZ

Smoky quartz is a translucent grayish/brown quartz with natural irradiation. This form of quartz will initiate movement of the basic, primal forces of your body, allowing you to express your physical self better. Smoky quartz will lend a person a sense of pride to be able to walk the Earth and inhabit a human body. It is very helpful for those of an earthy nature, and when worn as an amulet it can induce mental clarity and stimulate physical energy. It also protects and strengthens one while walking on the Earth.

SNOWFLAKE OBSIDIAN

Snowflake obsidian is a striking black, lustrous opaque stone with grayish/white bold markings, much like the beautiful patterns of snowflakes on a black background. It is a form of volcanic, amorphous, siliceous glassy rock. This form of obsidian is found in Utah.

Snowflake obsidian is said to sharpen both the external and the internal vision. It is one of the most important "teachers" of the New Age stones. It is the warrior of truth, and shows the self where the ego is at, and what it must change in order to advance to the next step of evolutionary growth.

With black on one end of the color scale and white on the other, we are shown the contrast of life: day and night, darkness and light, good and evil. The black symbolizes mastery over the physical plane, and the white symbolizes the purity inherent in each one of us. The snowflake obsidian helps to clear out cobwebs in the mind.

SNOW QUARTZ

Snow quartz is a delicate, translucent white form of quartz. It is a member of the chalcedony family, and is made of silica. It is a cryptocrystalline quartz and is found in Brazil, U.S. and Mexico.

Snow quartz helps us to have a focus of purity in ourselves. It helps for clarity of mind, and activates the crown chakra. It shows us our personal identification with the Infinite, the oneness with God. It represents peace and wisdom.

It is a stone that has the power to act as an insulator for all things. It can stop negative vibrations and maintain positive vibrations. Snow quartz can help develop psychic abilities. It causes the intellect to become more spiritual and helps one to have a love of truth.

SODALITE

Sodalite is a deep, rich blue stone with white inclusions. It is composed of chloric sodium aluminum silicate. It is found mostly in Canada and Brazil.

Sodalite is said to prolong physical endurance, and is used by athletes. It is said to help create harmony within the inner being and to stop conflict between the conscious mind and the subconscious. It is good for those who are oversensitive and reactive, allowing a person to shift from emotional to rational thinking. Sodalite helps clear away old mental patterns.

It helps one to understand the nature of one's self in relation to the universe. It awakens the third eye which prepares the mind to receive the inner light and intuitive knowledge. Sodalite is the densest and the most grounded of the deep blue stones, and clears the mind so that it can think with greater perception.

TIGER EYE

Tiger eye is a beautiful, golden-brown shiny stone which appears lifelike due to its chatoyancy, or silky luster. It is a crystallized quartz, made of silica. It is found mostly in Africa.

This stone has been worn through the ages to avert the evil eye and help prevent eye diseases. Tiger eye helps people gain insight into their own faults, and to think more clearly. This stone is helpful for greater spiritual understanding. It helps develop courage and inner strength, and gives one a sense of responsibility.

Tiger eye helps to defeat negative forces. Because of its ever-changing appearance when viewed from different angles, it helps the person using it to become "all seeing", able to view different ways of observing a situation. It gives one the ability to become more direct, more channeled in their way of thinking.

TOURMALINATED QUARTZ

Tourmalinated quartz is a clear form of quartz with silver filaments and threads of black tourmaline running through it. Much of this stone is found in Brazil.

Tourmalinated quartz is good for dissolving fear in oneself. It can aid in eliminating negative conditioning patterns we have experienced in our lives. Use of this type of quartz kept near the body and meditated upon is said to increase mental awareness and enhance psychic ability. It soothes the central nervous system, and helps to alleviate depression and nervous exhaustion. Because tourmalinated quartz is a combination of quartz and tourmaline, it has influences and characteristics of both these gems.

UNIKITE

Unikite is a combination of salmon pink feldspar and green epidote, and is an opaque stone. It is named after the Unikite Mountains between North Carolina and Tennessee, where it is found.

The pink in unikite speaks to the heart chakra to awaken the love within. The green lends it healing qualities to any hurts which have been sustained. The pink in unikite is a deeper shade of pink and is more grounding than that found in rose quartz. This stone has a leveling affect, and helps to balance the emotional aspects of the body. It is an earthy, peaceful stone.

CONCLUSION

The use of any form of quartz crystal will benefit you. What can you do with these gemstones and crystals to help yourself? Meditate with them. Place them on a part of your body that needs healing. Carry them around in your pocket. Wear them as jewelry or use them as a keychain. Sleep with them under your pillow. Put them on your desk, kitchen table, coffee table, anywhere that you will be near them and enjoy the benefits of their vibrations. They are just like a good friend—one whose companionship you delight in. Love them. Look at them. Enjoy them. They help you by their very presence. It's a gift they freely and lovingly give to you.

STAY IN TOUCH

On the following page you will find some of the books now available on related subjects. Your book dealer stocks most of these and will stock new titles in the Llewellyn series as they become available. We urge your patronage.

To obtain our full catalog write for our bimonthly news magazine/catalog, *Llewellyn's New Worlds of Mind and Spirit*. A sample copy is free, and it will continue coming to you at no cost as long as you are an active mail customer. Or you may subscribe for just $10.00 in the U.S.A. and Canada ($20.00 overseas, first class mail). Many bookstores also have *New Worlds* available to their customers. Ask for it.

Llewellyn's New Worlds of Mind and Spirit
P.O. Box 64383-360, St. Paul, MN 55164-0383, U.S.A.

TO ORDER BOOKS AND TAPES

If your book dealer does not have the books described, you may order them directly from the publisher by sending full price in U.S. funds, plus $3.00 for postage and handling for orders *under* $10.00; $4.00 for orders *over* $10.00. There are no postage and handling charges for orders over $50.00. Postage and handling rates are subject to change. We ship UPS whenever possible. Delivery guaranteed. Provide your street address as UPS does not deliver to P.O. Boxes. UPS to Canada requires a $50.00 minimum order. Allow 4-6 weeks for delivery. Orders outside the U.S.A. and Canada: Airmail—add retail price of book; add $5.00 for each non-book item (tapes, etc.); add $1.00 per item for surface mail. Mail orders to:

LLEWELLYN PUBLICATIONS
P.O. Box 64383-360, St. Paul, MN 55164-0383, U.S.A.

THE MESSAGE OF THE CRYSTAL SKULL
By Alice Bryant & Phyllis Galde

The most fascinating, mysterious artifact ever unearthed. Thousands of years old, yet it is beyond the capabilities of today's technology to duplicate it. Those who have touched the skull or seen photographs of it claim increased psychic abilities and purification. Read this book and discover how this mystical quartz crystal skull can benefit you and all of humankind. Famed bio-crystallographer Frank Dorland shares his research of the skull.

0-87542-092-3, 200 pgs., ills., photos, mass mrkt. $3.95

CRYSTAL AWARENESS
by Catherine Bowman

For millions of years, crystals have been waiting for people to discover their wonderful powers. Today they are used in watches, computer chips and communication devices. But there is also a spiritual holistic aspect to crystals.

Crystal Awareness will teach you everything you need to know about crystals to begin working with them. It will also help those who have been working with them to complete their knowledge.

Crystal Awareness is destined to be the guide of choice for people who are beginning their investigation of crystals:

0-87542-058-3, 200 pgs., illus., mass market $3.95